HEALTHY EATING TO PREVENT CANCER

Cancer-free Cookbook

Blake M. Davis

TABLE OF CONTENTS

INTRODUCTION

The prevalence of cancer has been rising over time, making it a major cause of death worldwide. A healthy lifestyle and the appropriate dietary choices can help lower the risk of acquiring cancer, even if there is no foolproof method of prevention. The "Healthy Eating To Prevent Cancer," a thorough manual on healthy diet and lifestyle choices that can help prevent cancer, comes into play here.

This cookbook offers a selection of mouthwatering dishes that are healthful and nutritious, all of which have been chosen to support a healthy lifestyle and avoid cancer. Using straightforward components that are easily found in grocery stores, the recipes are made to be simple to make. For sustaining a healthy diet and way of life, the book also offers professional guidance and useful tips.
More details on cancer risk factors and cancer prevention.

This book is a crucial tool for anybody interested in cancer prevention through nutrition and lifestyle, regardless of whether they want to make healthy lifestyle changes or have a personal or family history of the disease. You can take actions to lower your risk of cancer and live a healthier, happier life by adopting the ideas presented in this book into your everyday practice.

When given a cancer diagnosis, many people experience fear and helplessness. Although cancer prevention may seem like a difficult endeavor, it's vital to keep in mind that even the smallest modification in your lifestyle can significantly lower your risk. You may learn a ton about dietary and lifestyle decisions that can help prevent cancer in "Healthy eating to prevent cancer," which is a goldmine of knowledge. Fruits and vegetables, whole grains, and healthy fats are just a few of the food types and nutrients that are broken down into chapters in the book. In addition to a list of scrumptious and nutritious dishes that use these components, each chapter contains an explanation of the advantages of these foods.

The dishes in this cookbook are delicious and simple to prepare, in addition to being intended to encourage cancer prevention. Every meal, from salads and smoothies to main courses and desserts, is painstakingly created to be both nourishing and enticing. In addition, the book offers advice on how to plan meals, buy for groceries, and further way of life adjustments that can help to ensure a healthy and cancer-free lifetime.

In the end, "Healthy Eating To Prevent Cancer" is much more than simply a cookbook; it's a thorough manual for leading a healthier and happier life. You can lower your risk of cancer and enhance your general health and well-being by choosing the appropriate food and lifestyle. Therefore "Healthy Eating To Prevent Cancer" is the ideal resource for you, whether you're trying to avoid cancer or just want to make healthy decisions every day.

CHAPTER ONE

UNDERSTANDING THE CONNECTION BETWEEN DIET AND CANCER

Millions of people around the world suffer from cancer each year, which is a terrible disease. It is becoming increasingly obvious that there are complex and multifactorial causes of the disease as cancer incidence rises despite significant technological advancements in medicine. The relationship between diet and cancer is one research topic that has attracted more attention recently. We will look at the evidence for this connection in this chapter of the book and discuss how it may affect the diagnosis and treatment of cancer.
A vast variety of nutrients are necessary for the efficient operation of the human body, which is a complicated system. Our main supply of essential nutrients comes from the food we consume, and this has a significant influence on our health and happiness. So, it is not unexpected that research on the connection between nutrition and cancer is gaining popularity. There is currently a substantial body of research that suggests

our diet has a big impact on our chance of getting cancer.

Obesity is one of the dietary elements most clearly linked to a higher risk of cancer. Breast, colon, and prostate cancer are just a few of the cancers for which obesity is a major risk factor.The connection between obesity and cancer is thought to be caused, at least in part, by the fact that adipose tissue releases hormones and other signaling molecules that can encourage the growth of cancer cells. Moreover, obesity is frequently linked to other harmful lifestyle elements, such as a bad diet and insufficient exercise, which can raise the risk of cancer even higher.

The consumption of processed and red meat is a significant contributor to the relationship between diet and cancer. According to a number of studies, eating a lot of processed and red meat increases the risk of getting numerous cancers, including colorectal, pancreatic, and prostate cancer. Although the cause of this connection is unclear, it is believed to be connected to the presence of carcinogenic chemicals that are created during the processing and cooking of meat.

There is proof that particular nutrients and dietary habits help prevent cancer in addition to these dietary factors. For instance, numerous studies have revealed that diets rich in fruits, vegetables, and whole grains are linked to a lower risk of multiple cancer types, such as breast, colorectal, and lung cancer. Certain foods are a good source of antioxidants and other substances that can shield cells from harm and stop the spread of cancer cells.Omega-3 fatty acids, which are present in fatty fish and specific kinds of nuts and seeds, as well as tea, which has chemicals with anti-inflammatory and antioxidant effects, are other dietary elements that have been demonstrated to have a protective impact against cancer. Additionally, a number of studies have demonstrated that fasting or calorie restriction can lower the risk of cancer by encouraging cellular repair and lowering inflammation.

We still know very little about the precise processes by which nutrition impacts cancer development, despite the expanding body of evidence linking diet to cancer risk. Also, it's critical to remember that cancer is a complicated illness with a variety of causes.Therefore, it is improbable that a single dietary element will be the only contributor to cancer. Yet, the data do support the notion that altering one's diet might be a useful tactic for lowering the risk of cancer and enhancing general health.

Moreover, it should be noted that the connection between nutrition and cancer is a complicated and diverse subject that calls for more investigation. The research does, however, point to the fact that consuming fewer processed meats and more lean proteins while keeping a balanced diet rich in a range of fruits, vegetables, whole grains, and lean proteins can greatly lower the risk of several cancers. We may take an active role in lowering our risk of cancer development and enhancing our general health and wellbeing by making little modifications to our diets.

CHAPTER TWO

FUNCTION OF IMPORTANT FOODS AND NUTRIENTS IN FOSTERING CELLULAR HEALTH AND IMMUNITY

With an anticipated 19.3 million new instances of cancer and 10 million cancer-related deaths reported in 2020, cancer is still the leading cause of mortality and morbidity worldwide. Although cancer is a complicated and multifaceted disease, new research indicates that diet and nutrition may be crucial in preventing cancer by affecting cellular metabolism, oxidative stress, inflammation, and DNA damage. This chapter will review the multidisciplinary science of cancer prevention and look at the role that certain foods and minerals can play in boosting cellular health and immunity.

First Section

Introduction To Cancer Biology.

The biology of cancer, including the cellular and molecular processes that underlie the onset and spread of the disease, will be briefly discussed in this section. We'll talk about the fundamental biological pathways that control cell growth, division, and death, as well as the roles that genetic mutations, epigenetic changes, and environmental variables play in the development of cancer. Aspects such as immune surveillance, immune evasion, and immunotherapy will all be covered in our discussion of the immune system's function in cancer prevention and treatment.

The aberrant cellular growth and division that causes cancer is a complex disease. The biology of cancer will be briefly discussed in this section, along with the mechanisms that explain the growth and spread of the disease.

Genetic alterations are one of the main causes of the development of cancer. These mutations may develop naturally or may be brought on by a number of different things, including exposure to radiation or specific chemicals. Important genes that control cell growth, division, and death, as well as their expression, can be affected by genetic abnormalities, which can result in unchecked cellular proliferation.

Cancer development is also greatly influenced by epigenetic alterations, which are changes in gene expression without corresponding changes in the underlying DNA sequence. These alterations can activate oncogenes, mutate chromatin structure, and quiet tumor-suppressing genes, all of which help cancer cells grow and survive.

Cancer development can also be influenced by environmental elements like smoking, UV radiation exposure, and specific diseases. These elements have the potential to deteriorate DNA and set off genetic changes, which can result in the beginning and development of cancer.

The regulation of cell growth, division, and death involves a number of biological pathways, including the PI3K/AKT/mTOR, MAPK/ERK, and TP53 pathways. Dysregulation of these pathways can encourage the growth of cancer by enabling cells to evade regular cell cycle checkpoints and multiply uncontrolled.
A crucial part of preventing and treating cancer is played by the immune system. Prior to the formation of a tumor, the immune system can identify and destroy cancer cells thanks to the immune surveillance mechanism. Yet, there are a number of ways in which cancer cells can avoid being recognized and eliminated by the immune system. These include suppressing the production of antigens and creating immunosuppressive substances.

Enhancing the immune system's capacity to identify and destroy cancer cells is the goal of the potential cancer treatment method known as immunotherapy. Checkpoint inhibitors and chimeric antigen receptor (CAR) T-cell therapy are two examples of several immunotherapy modalities that have demonstrated promising outcomes in the treatment of specific cancers.

In conclusion, implementing successful prevention and treatment plans for this disease depends on having a solid grasp of the biology of cancer. For the creation of targeted medicines and immunotherapies, it is crucial to understand the cellular and molecular mechanisms behind cancer growth and progression, including genetic mutations, epigenetic alterations, environmental variables, cellular pathways, and immune system control.

Section Two

The Function Of Nutrients In The Prevention Of Cancer

The role of important nutrients in preventing cancer will be the main topic of this section. We'll look at the epidemiological and clinical data demonstrating how certain nutrients and food components, like vitamins, minerals, antioxidants, fiber, and phytochemicals, can lower the chance of developing cancer. We will also go through the underlying cellular and molecular processes of these nutrients' anticancer actions, such as their control of oxidative stress, DNA damage, and inflammation.

Genetics, way of life, and environmental variables are only a few of the many risk factors for cancer. Nutrition is a crucial component of cancer prevention, and studies have shown that some nutrients can significantly lower the risk of developing cancer.
Important nutrients that have been demonstrated to be helpful in lowering the risk of cancer include vitamins, minerals, antioxidants, fiber, and phytochemicals. Consuming particular minerals and food components has been associated with a lower risk of cancer by epidemiological and clinical studies.

Vitamins like vitamin A, vitamin C, and vitamin E are well known for their antioxidant capabilities, which help shield the body against oxidative stress and inflammation, both of which can aid in the development of cancer. Also, it has been demonstrated that specific B-vitamins, such as folate, can aid in the prevention of cancers like colon and breast cancer.
There is evidence that certain cancers are less likely to develop when minerals like calcium and selenium are consumed. In contrast to selenium, which has been associated to a lower incidence of prostate cancer, calcium aids in the prevention of colon cancer.

The category of nutrients known as antioxidants is another crucial one for preventing cancer. They include phytochemicals like flavonoids, beta-carotene, and lycopene, which are present in fruits, vegetables, and other plant-based diets. Oxidative stress, which can harm cells and promote the growth of cancer, is something that antioxidants shield the body against.

In addition to maintaining digestive health and possibly lowering the incidence of colon cancer, fiber is crucial for cancer prevention. Fruits, vegetables, whole grains, and legumes are just a few of the foods that contain fiber. Plant-based substances known as phytochemicals have been found to have anti-cancer effects. They include compounds like curcumin, which is present in turmeric, and resveratrol, which can be found in red wine and grapes. By lowering inflammation, encouraging healthy cell growth, and guarding against oxidative stress and DNA damage, phytochemicals have been demonstrated to help prevent cancer.

It is critical to comprehend the underlying cellular and molecular mechanisms by which certain nutrients exert their anti-cancer benefits in addition to looking at the epidemiological and clinical evidence that links these nutrients and food components to a decreased risk of developing cancer. For instance, a lot of these nutrients can control DNA damage, oxidative stress, and inflammation, all of which contribute to the growth of cancer.

Conclusion: While no single nutrient or food will completely prevent cancer, a diet high in vitamins, minerals, antioxidants, fiber, and phytochemicals can help to lower the risk of cancer. People can minimize their chance of developing cancer by making educated decisions about their food and lifestyle choices by understanding the function that these nutrients play in cancer prevention.

Section Three

Nutritional Habits And Cancer Prevention

We will look at the connection between eating habits and cancer prevention in this part. We'll look at the data demonstrating how certain eating habits, such as the Mediterranean diet, the DASH diet, and the plant-based diet, reduce the chance of developing cancer. We will also talk about possible processes by which certain dietary practices have anti-cancer effects immunity and inflammation.

Genetics, environmental exposures, and lifestyle decisions are just a few of the variables that might have an impact on the complicated disease of cancer. Diet has been identified as a significant modifiable risk factor for cancer among various lifestyle factors. Researchers have studied the effect of various food patterns on cancer risk over time, and mounting data suggests that some dietary patterns may be protective against cancer.

The Mediterranean diet is one of the dietary regimens that has received the most research about cancer prevention. This eating style is defined by a high intake of plant-based foods, such as fruits, vegetables, whole grains, legumes, nuts, and seeds, combined with fish, olive oil, and moderate amounts of dairy, poultry, and red wine.According to a number of studies, following a Mediterranean diet may lower your chance of developing cancer, including breast, colorectal, and prostate cancer. The Mediterranean diet's capacity to support a healthy gut flora as well as its high level of fiber, antioxidants, and anti-inflammatory substances may be responsible for its preventive effects.

The DASH (Dietary Approaches to Stop Hypertension) diet is another eating regimen that has been demonstrated to lower cancer risk. This eating style is high in fruits, vegetables, whole grains, lean protein, and low-fat dairy, while being low in saturated and trans fats, added sweets, and sodium. A lower risk of numerous malignancies, such as colorectal, breast, and lung cancer, has been associated with the DASH diet.Due to its capacity to lower oxidative stress, inflammation, and insulin resistance—all of which are linked to the development of cancer—the DASH diet may have a positive impact on cancer risk.

A lower risk of cancer has also been linked to plant-based diets that prioritize the consumption of fruits, vegetables, whole grains, legumes, nuts, and seeds while limiting or avoiding animal products. A substantial body of research indicates that plant-based diets may lower the incidence of various cancer types, including colon, breast, and prostate cancer. Plant-based diets' propensity to influence cellular metabolism and support a healthy gut flora, as well as their high concentrations of phytochemicals, fiber, and antioxidants, may be to blame for their anti-cancer properties.

The research suggests that eating habits are crucial in the fight against cancer. Commitment to a healthy, balanced diet with an emphasis on plant-based foods, whole grains, lean protein, and healthy fats while reducing processed and red meat, sugar, and sodium is probably going to provide protection against cancer. The Mediterranean diet, the DASH diet, and plant-based diets are just a few of the various eating regimens covered in this section that have all been linked to a lower risk of cancer and may provide useful dietary advice for cancer prevention. It is necessary to conduct more study to develop more focused dietary treatments for cancer prevention and to better understand the processes through which certain dietary patterns exert their anti-cancer effects.

Section Four

Integrative Cancer Prevention Strategies

The use of dietary supplements, functional foods, and complementary and alternative medicine are among integrative methods for cancer prevention that will be covered in this section. In this section, we'll look at the research proving that some supplements, like vitamin D, omega-3 fatty acids, and probiotics, can prevent cancer. We will also go over any potential dangers, restrictions, and combinations with other cancer treatments that may come with using these supplements.

A thorough strategy is necessary for cancer prevention because it is a complicated and diverse problem. Integrative methods, which mix conventional and alternative medicines, can also be successful in lowering the risk of cancer, even if traditional medicine plays a crucial role in cancer prevention. We'll look at a few integrative methods for preventing cancer in this part, such as using functional foods, dietary supplements, and complementary and alternative therapies.

As a way to lower the chance of developing cancer, dietary supplements are growing in popularity. Probiotics, vitamin D, and omega-3 fatty acids are some of the most often utilized supplements in the fight against cancer. Many forms of cancer can be prevented by consuming enough vitamin D, which is an essential nutrient.stomach cancer in color. Vitamin D has been found to assist control cell growth and stop the growth of cancerous cells, according to studies. Omega-3 fatty acids, which are present in fatty fish, can lower the risk of cancer by lowering inflammatory responses in the body. Probiotics, which are healthy bacteria that live in the gut, can help prevent cancer by enhancing gut health and lowering inflammation.

While some studies have suggested that dietary supplements may be effective in preventing cancer, there are also potential hazards and restrictions related to their usage. High dosages of some supplements, for instance, can be detrimental and potentially raise the risk of developing cancer. Furthermore, some supplements may interact with common cancer therapies like chemotherapy and radiation therapy, which may lessen their efficacy or result in negative side effects.

Although some studies have suggested that dietary supplements may be effective in preventing cancer, there are also potential hazards and restrictions related to their usage. For instance, taking certain supplements in large doses might be dangerous and even raise your risk of developing cancer. Moreover, some supplements may interact negatively or ineffectively with common cancer therapies including chemotherapy and radiation therapy. Functional foods, which are foods that have been demonstrated to have certain health advantages, can be utilized in conjunction with dietary supplements as part of an integrative approach to cancer prevention. Examples of foods that have been proven to have anti-cancer qualities include the cruciferous veggies broccoli and cauliflower. Green tea, which possesses antioxidants, has also been demonstrated to have anti-cancer effects. An integrative strategy to prevent cancer might also include the use of complementary and alternative medicine (CAM) treatments including acupuncture, massage, and meditation. While there isn't enough data to prove that these treatments are useful at preventing cancer, some studies have found that they can help people manage their stress levels, enhance their quality

of life, and manage symptoms related to cancer and
cancer treatments.

CHAPTER THREE

SUPERFOODS THAT CAN HELP PREVENT CANCER

Berries: Antioxidants found in berries help shield the body's cells from damage brought on by free radicals. Great choices include blackberries, blueberries, raspberries, and strawberries.

Cruciferous vegetables: Foods high in glucosinolates, which have been demonstrated to aid in the prevention and treatment of cancer, include broccoli, cauliflower, kale, and Brussels sprouts.

Tomatoes: Lycopene, a potent antioxidant that has been demonstrated to aid in the prevention of cancer, is abundant in tomatoes.

Garlic: Sulfur compounds found in garlic, which may help lower the incidence of some malignancies like colon and stomach cancer.

Turmeric: Curcumin, a substance found in turmeric, is anti-inflammatory and antioxidant, and it may have cancer-preventive effects.

Green tea: Green tea contains a high concentration of catechins, an antioxidant that can thwart the formation of cancer cells and combat free radicals.

Nuts: Healthy fats, protein, and fiber can all be found in nuts. Moreover, they include phytochemicals and antioxidants that may help lower the risk of cancer.

Fatty fish: Omega-3 fatty acids, found in abundance in fatty fish like salmon, mackerel, and sardines, have been demonstrated to have anti-inflammatory qualities and may help lower the risk of cancer.

Lentils and Beans: Lentils and beans are wonderful sources of fiber, protein, and other nutrients that may help prevent cancer
Dark leafy greens: Vegetables and fruits high in vitamins, minerals, and antioxidants, such as spinach, kale, and collard greens, may help lower the risk of cancer.

Citrus fruits: Citrus fruits, such as oranges, lemons, and grapefruits, are rich in vitamin C, a potent antioxidant that may help prevent cancer.

Whole grains: Grains such as brown rice, quinoa, and whole wheat are excellent sources of fiber and other nutrients that may help lower the risk of cancer.

Mushrooms: Mushrooms include substances called polysaccharides that may strengthen the immune system and have anti-cancer qualities.

Sweet Potatoes: Beta-carotene, an antioxidant that may aid in cancer prevention, is abundant in sweet potatoes.

Yogurt: Yogurt has probiotics, which are good bacteria that may assist the immune system and lessen inflammation while also possibly lowering the risk of cancer.

Although several spices have been investigated for their potential anti-cancer properties, it's crucial to remember that no one food or spice may cause cancer or cure it. But adding a variety of spices to a healthy diet may have some advantages for your health. Following are some spices whose potential to prevent cancer have been researched:

Turmeric: Curcumin, the main compound in turmeric, has been investigated for its possible anti-inflammatory and antioxidant properties, which may help prevent the onset of cancer.

Ginger: Studies have demonstrated the anti-inflammatory and antioxidant benefits of substances found in ginger such as gingerols and shogaols. Studies have suggested that ginger may have anti-cancer properties.

Cinnamon: Many substances found in cinnamon, such as cinnamaldehyde, cinnamic acid, and cinnamate, may have anti-inflammatory and antioxidant benefits. Cinnamon may potentially have cancer-fighting benefits, according to some research.

Garlic: This vegetable includes sulfur compounds that may have anti-cancer properties. Consuming garlic may help lower your chance of developing some cancers, such as colorectal and stomach cancer, according to several studies.

Black pepper: Studies have demonstrated the anti-inflammatory and antioxidant properties of piperine, the primary component in black pepper. According to certain research, piperine might have anti-cancer potential.

Despite the fact that certain spices may have health advantages, further research is necessary to completely comprehend their anti-cancer properties and how they might be used in cancer prevention and treatment programs.

For their culinary and therapeutic benefits, spices have been utilized for thousands of years. Interest in the potential anti-cancer properties of several spices has grown over the past few years. Spices may have a number of health advantages, including potential anti-cancer characteristics, according to some studies, though more research is required to fully understand the processes underlying these effects.

Turmeric is one of the spices that has been the most thoroughly researched for its possible anti-cancer properties. There is evidence that the primary component of turmeric, curcumin, has anti-inflammatory, characteristics that fight cancer and act as antioxidants. Curcumin may be able to stop the growth and spread of some malignancies, including breast, colon, and pancreatic cancer, according to some research.

The possible anti-cancer properties of ginger have also been investigated. It has been demonstrated that the anti-inflammatory and antioxidant effects of ginger's constituents, gingerols and shogaols, are present. According to several research, ginger may be able to stop the growth and recurrence of a few cancers, including colon and ovarian cancer.

The anti-cancer effects of cinnamon are also potentially present in other spices. A number of the substances found in cinnamon, such as cinnamaldehyde, cinnamic

acid, and cinnamate, may have anti-inflammatory and antioxidant properties.
Some diseases, such as leukemia and colorectal cancer, may be able to be halted in their tracks before they even begin, according to certain research.

The possible anti-cancer properties of garlic have also been investigated. Sulfur molecules found in garlic might be able to fight cancer. Consuming garlic may help lower your chance of developing some cancers, such as colorectal and stomach cancer, according to several studies.

An additional spice that may be healthy is black pepper, which may also have anti-cancer qualities. The active component of black pepper, piperine, has been demonstrated to have anti-inflammatory and antioxidant properties. According to some studies, piperine may aid in the prevention of the growth and metastasis of some cancers, such as breast and lung cancer.

It's crucial to remember that no one item or spice will prevent or cure cancer on its own, even while including certain spices in a balanced diet may give possible health benefits. A balanced diet high in fruits, vegetables, whole grains, lean proteins, and healthy fats, regular exercise, and abstaining from cigarettes and excessive alcohol consumption are crucial steps for lowering the risk of cancer and maintaining general health.

Curcumin, a substance found in turmeric, has been investigated for its anti-inflammatory and antioxidant properties. According to certain research, curcumin may aid in the prevention of some cancers, including colon, breast, and prostate cancer.

Garlic: Studies have indicated that the sulfur compounds found in garlic have anticancer properties. Garlic may help prevent colorectal and stomach cancer, according to some research.

Ginger: Research has shown that the chemicals gingerols and shogaols in ginger have anti-inflammatory and antioxidant properties. According to certain research, ginger may help protect against some cancers, including ovarian and colorectal cancer.

Green tea: Green tea includes substances known as catechins, which have been found to have antioxidant and anti-inflammatory benefits. Many cancers, including breast, prostate, and colorectal cancer, may be prevented by green tea, according to certain research.

Milk thistle: Silymarin, a substance found in milk thistle that has been investigated for possible anti-cancer properties, is present in the plant. According to certain research, silymarin may be useful in preventing some cancers, such as liver cancer.

In order to properly comprehend the potential advantages and hazards of utilizing these herbs for cancer prevention, it is crucial to keep in mind that more research is required. While utilizing herbs to prevent cancer, it is always advisable to see a healthcare professional first.

CHAPTER FOUR

BASICS COOKING TOOLS AND EQUIPMENT FOR CANCER-FREE KITCHEN

Millions of individuals worldwide have been impacted by the terrible disease of cancer. A number of things, including genetics, way of life, and exposure to the environment, can contribute to this complex illness. There are various ways to lower the risk of getting cancer, even if there is no single treatment that will cure it. Creating a kitchen free of cancer is one such step, and it involves employing necessary cooking appliances and instruments that can assist in stopping the creation of substances that can cause cancer in food.

No amount of emphasis can be placed enough on the necessity of creating a cancer-free kitchen. By choosing a healthy lifestyle, it has been demonstrated that up to 40% of cancer cases can be avoided.

Cooking techniques can be extremely important in lowering the incidence of cancer, and the food we consume can have a big impact on our health.

Investing in top-notch cooking supplies and equipments is the first step in creating a kitchen free of cancer. Cookware made of stainless steel, cast iron, or ceramic is a fantastic choice because they are non-reactive and do not contaminate food with dangerous substances. When heated to high temperatures, non-stick cookware can emit poisonous vapors, thus it should be avoided.

A high-quality blender is yet another crucial appliance for a cancer-free kitchen. The body may more easily absorb nutrients when fruits and vegetables are blended to help break down cell walls. Moreover, food cancer-causing chemicals can be lessened by blending.

A cancer-free kitchen must have healthy products in addition to culinary supplies. A balanced diet should be built on a foundation of fresh produce, complete grains, lean protein, and healthy fats. As organic food is free of dangerous pesticides and other chemicals that increase the risk of cancer, it is advised.

A cancer-free kitchen is built using cooking techniques that are important. Carcinogens are substances that can cause cancer, and they can be produced by grilling, frying, and broiling. Cooking techniques that don't produce toxic substances, such as steaming, boiling, and baking, are advised instead.

The temperature at which food is being cooked should also be carefully monitored. It is advised to cook food at lower temperatures for a longer period of time because cooking at high temperatures might lead to the development of hazardous substances. Creating a cancer-free kitchen should focus on slow cooking techniques like those that use a crockpot or pressure cooker.

A food processor, a vegetable steamer, and a water filter are further appliances that can support a kitchen without cancer. Healthy dips and spreads can be made using a food processor, and heating veggies in a vegetable steamer can help preserve their nutrients. From tap water, which can be a substantial source of exposure to dangerous chemicals, a water filter can eliminate harmful impurities.

The ingredients and meals we use when cooking also play a role in creating a cancer-free kitchen. It's crucial to select foods that are both nutrient-dense and free of hazardous ingredients. For instance, foods high in antioxidants, like blueberries and leafy greens, can help stave against cancer-causing free radicals. Other significant sources of fiber and nutrients that can support overall health include whole grains like quinoa and brown rice.

Reduced intake of packaged and processed foods is a crucial factor to take into account when designing a cancer-free kitchen. These foods frequently have high concentrations of additives, preservatives, and other substances that can raise the risk of cancer.

Choose fresh, healthy meals that have not been overly processed and are devoid of dangerous substances.

Considering how we cook and preserve our food is also crucial. For instance, cooking or heating food in plastic containers might cause dangerous chemicals to leak into the food. Utilizing glass or stainless steel containers can be a safer choice. Also, washing fruits and vegetables properly can aid in getting rid of any remaining pesticides or other toxins.

It's crucial to select cooking oils that are both low in hazardous chemicals and stable at high temperatures. Olive oil, avocado oil, and coconut oil are all suitable substitutes.Conversely, it is best to stay away from vegetable oils that are high in omega-6 fatty acids because they can cause inflammation and raise the risk of cancer. Examples of these oils are corn oil and soybean oil.

It's crucial to restrict alcohol intake and the use of processed meats, both of which have been linked to an increased risk of cancer. Healthy ingredients and cooking techniques are also key. Limit your intake of red meat to once a week or fewer and choose lean protein sources like chicken, fish, and lentils in its place.

In conclusion, creating a cancer-free kitchen requires making wise decisions regarding the appliances and tools we employ, the products we cook with, and the manner in which we prepare our meals. We can lessen the risk of cancer and enhance general health and wellbeing by consuming healthy, whole foods and cooking them according to suggested techniques. On our health and the health of those around us, even even minor changes can have a significant influence.

Chapter Five

THE ESSENTIALS FOR HEALTHY COOKING

For great, wholesome meals to be made at home, your pantry must be stocked with the necessary components. You won't have to run to the grocery store every day if your pantry is well-stocked because you'll be able to prepare healthy meals quickly. We'll go over all the items you need to stock up on in this book chapter so that your pantry is always stocked with everything you need to prepare wholesome meals.

Let's start by discussing grains in the first place. Grains are an essential component of a balanced diet and a versatile food that can be utilized in many different recipes. Options such as whole-grain pasta, brown rice, quinoa, and oats are excellent.The variety of whole-grain pasta available is fantastic. They are loaded with important nutrients including vitamins, minerals, and antioxidants and are high in fiber, which can help you feel content and full.

Legumes have a low fat content and are a great source of fiber and plant-based protein. It's a good idea to stock your cupboard with lentils, chickpeas, black beans, and kidney beans. They can be used to add flavor and texture to a variety of dishes, including soups, stews, salads, and wraps.

Nuts and seeds are another important component of healthy cooking. Healthy fats, protein, and fiber are all abundant in nuts and seeds. The best options to have on hand are almonds, cashews, walnuts, and sunflower seeds. They are a fantastic ingredient to have on hand for snacks when you need a quick energy boost and can be used in a range of dishes, from granola to trail mix.

Moreover, a healthy pantry must have spices and herbs. They're a wonderful way to flavor your food without adding extra fat or sodium. It's a good idea to have spices on hand such as cumin, turmeric, ginger, and garlic. Antioxidants and anti-inflammatory qualities found in them are abundant, and they may improve general health and wellbeing.
Oils and vinegars are additional key components for healthy cooking. When it comes to cooking oils, coconut oil, avocado oil, and olive oil are all excellent choices. They can support heart health because they contain a lot of heart-healthy fats. When preparing dressings or marinades, red wine vinegar, apple cider vinegar, and balsamic vinegar are all excellent choices. They're a fantastic way to flavor your food without adding extra fat or sugar.

Along with these essential ingredients, it's crucial to keep a variety of fruits and vegetables on hand. A healthy diet should include plenty of fresh produce because it gives food flavor and nutrition.

Nuts and seeds are another important component of healthy cooking. Healthy fats, protein, and fiber are all abundant in nuts and seeds. The best options to have on hand are almonds, cashews, walnuts, and sunflower seeds. They are a fantastic ingredient to have on hand for snacks when you need a quick energy boost and can be used in a range of dishes, from granola to trail mix.

Moreover, a healthy pantry must have spices and herbs. They're a wonderful way to flavor your food without adding extra fat or salt. It's a good idea to have spices on hand such as cumin, turmeric, ginger, and garlic. Antioxidants and anti-inflammatory qualities found in them are abundant, and they may improve general health and wellbeing.

Oils and vinegars are additional key ingredients for wholesome cooking. The three oils that are best to use when cooking are coconut, avocado, and olive. These are heart-healthy foods with a lot of good fats. When preparing dressings or marinades, apple cider vinegar, balsamic vinegar, and red wine vinegar are all excellent choices. They are a wonderful way to flavor your food without adding extra fat or sugar.

Having a variety of fruits and veggies on hand is equally as crucial as having these must-have items. A healthy diet must include fresh vegetables, which is also a delicious and nutritious way to enhance your meals.

An essential step in preparing delicious, nutrient-dense meals at home is stocking your pantry with essential components for healthy cooking. You won't have to run to the grocery store every day if your pantry is well-stocked because you'll be able to prepare healthy meals quickly. It's imperative to always have on hand ingredients like grains, legumes, nuts, seeds, spices, herbs, oils, vinegars, and fresh veggies. You'll be well on your way to cooking tasty, nutritious meals that you and your family will like if you stock your pantry with these products.

CHAPTER SIX

FOOD PREPARATION TO AVOID CANCER

A potent weapon in your toolbox to protect your health and wellbeing is meal planning for cancer prevention. It entails selecting and preparing foods that are high in nutrients and antioxidants while reducing your intake of hazardous ingredients like processed meats, sugar, and unhealthy fats.

You can lower your risk of developing cancer and other chronic diseases by planning your meals carefully and deliberately. Also, you can increase your energy levels, strengthen your immune system, and enhance your general quality of life.

So what does meal planning for cancer prevention look like? It begins with choosing a variety of healthy, plant-based foods such fruits, vegetables, whole grains, legumes, and nuts. These meals are teeming with fiber, vitamins, and minerals that support the strength and wellness of your body.

Also, since red and processed meats have been associated with an elevated risk of numerous types of cancer, it's crucial to limit your intake of these foods.

Instead, think about adding extra beans, lentils, tofu, and tempeh—plant-based protein sources—to your meals.

Focus on including healthful fats in your diet, such as olive oil, avocado, and almonds, while avoiding trans fats and saturated fats. Keep in mind that too much sugar can cause inflammation and otherwise health issues, so watch how much of it you consume.

It's important to ensure you are getting a variety of nutrients while meal planning for cancer prevention in addition to picking the correct foods. Consuming a rainbow of fruits and vegetables can help you acquire the varied phytonutrients, vitamins, and minerals your body needs to function correctly and fight cancer.

Regarding your meals' portion amounts, it's equally critical to pay attention. It is possible to gain weight and develop cancer if you consume too much of any food, even nutritious foods. Control your portion sizes in accordance with your goal of eating balanced meals that feature a range of foods.
Meal planning is not the only way to lower your risk of cancer; you can also lower your risk by planning regular physical activity into your daily schedule. A healthy weight can be maintained with exercise, which also strengthens the immune system and reduces body inflammation.

Consider speaking with a certified dietitian to help you design a personalized meal plan based on your unique needs and preferences if you are unsure of where to begin with meal planning for cancer prevention. They can also offer advice on how to shop wisely and choose healthful meals when dining out.

Remember that there is no one-size-fits-all strategy for meal preparation in the fight against cancer. Depending on your age, gender, lifestyle, and medical background, your demands may change.The secret is to prioritize consuming a range of nutrient-dense meals while minimizing your intake of processed foods, red and processed meats, and harmful fats and carbohydrates.

Meal planning for cancer prevention can be an effective technique to safeguard your health and wellbeing. You may lower your risk of getting cancer and maintain excellent health for years to come by intentionally choosing the foods you eat.

Chapter seven

BREAKFASTS TO START YOUR DAY

As the name suggests, breakfast is the meal that breaks the overnight fast and refuels the body with energy after a long night of sleep. With good reason, it is frequently referred to as the most significant meal of the day. Breakfast gives us the nutrients and energy we need to start the day, so it's critical to select wholesome foods that will keep us full and satisfied until our next meal while also giving us lasting energy.

Let's start off by discussing the advantages of eating a healthy breakfast in the morning. According to studies, those who regularly eat breakfast tend to be healthier overall, with lower rates of obesity, type 2 diabetes, and heart disease. A healthy breakfast can also help with cognitive function, memory, and concentration, making it simpler to concentrate on work or school assignments throughout the day. Additionally, breakfast can give us the nutrients we need to support muscle growth and repair. It can also help with weight management by lowering hunger and preventing overeating later in the day.

Given how crucial breakfast is, let's look at some nutritious and delectable options that might give us a good start to the day. The first item on our list is overnight oats, a quick but filling meal that can be made ahead of time and tailored to your taste preferences. Just combine rolled oats, milk or yogurt, and your preferred garnishes (such as nuts, fruit, or honey) in a jar or container and chill overnight. Your breakfast will be ready in the morning and will be creamy and tasty.

A smoothie bowl, which is simply a thicker version of a smoothie and is topped with various nutrient-dense ingredients like granola, fresh fruit, and nuts, is another fantastic breakfast choice.
Smoothie bowls may be readily adjusted to match your dietary demands and taste preferences and are not only tasty but also nutrient-rich.

Eggs are a fantastic alternative if you're searching for a more conventional morning food. Having a breakfast of eggs might help you feel full and satisfied throughout the morning because they are high in protein. Scrambled, fried, poached, or boiled are just a few of the countless egg preparation options. For a complete and well-balanced breakfast, add some whole-grain toast and fresh fruit on the side.

The traditional morning mainstay, oatmeal, is a must-have, too. Fiber from oatmeal is a fantastic source for promoting digestive health and lowering cholesterol. To add sweetness and taste, you can mix it with milk or water and top it with a variety of garnishes, such as nuts, fruit, or honey. Those who like a warm and cozy breakfast during the winter months have oatmeal as a terrific alternative.

Certainly! It can be overwhelming to choose from all the breakfast alternatives available. It is possible to cook wholesome, delectable breakfasts that will improve your mood, though, with a little forethought and preparation.

The balance of macronutrients, including protein, carbs, and fat, is a crucial consideration when deciding on breakfast selections. All three macronutrients should be consumed at breakfast to ensure a balanced breakfast that will keep your blood sugar levels stable and your hunger at bay. By way of illustration, including protein in your morning meal can aid in reducing cravings and preventing overeating later in the day. Yogurt, nut butter, eggs, and tofu are excellent sources of protein.
As a source of fuel and energy for the body, carbohydrates are very crucial. Complex carbs, which are strong in fiber and offer sustaining energy throughout the morning, should be chosen instead, such as whole grains, fruits, and vegetables. Steer clear of processed carbs like white bread and sugary cereals that can induce blood sugar dips and rises.

An ideal breakfast should include both healthy fats and carbohydrates. They support maintaining a sense of fullness and satisfaction and may even enhance cognitive performance. Olive oil, almonds, seeds, and avocados are excellent sources of good fats.

Aside from balancing your macronutrient intake, you need also think about the quality of the foods you consume.

Avoid highly processed and packaged foods, which are frequently filled with extra sugar and bad fats, and try to choose whole, less processed foods wherever you can.

water intake should not be overlooked. A glass of water can hydrate your body and enhance digestion when you start your day. To give your water even more flavor and nourishment, you may also add some lemon or cucumber slices.

Thee key to achieving your best level of health and wellbeing is to start each day with a nutritious breakfast that is balanced. Making energizing, filling breakfasts that will last you the entire day is simple with a little forethought and preparation. In order to select the breakfast option that is best for you and your body, try out a few different options.

Oatmeal is a traditional breakfast food that cannot be overlooked. Oatmeal is a fantastic source of fiber, which can help lower cholesterol and support digestive health. It can be made with milk or water and garnished with different items like nuts, fruit, or honey to add sweetness and flavor. For those who prefer a warm and cozy breakfast during the colder months, oatmeal is also a great choice.

CHAPTER EIGHT

CANCER-FIGHTING DESSERTS

A nutritious diet can be quite important in the fight against cancer. Despite the fact that desserts are frequently linked to indulgence and unhealthful eating patterns, there are many mouthwatering and nutritious options that can help prevent cancer. Here are a few suggestions for sweets that are nutritious and can help fight cancer:

Fruits are rich in elements that can help lower the risk of cancer, including antioxidants, so a fresh fruit salad is a great idea. An energizing and healthful dessert choice is a fruit salad in all different colors.

Even though it may sound strange, dark chocolate can be a nutritious dessert option. Having been proven to have anti-cancer qualities, dark chocolate is abundant in antioxidants.

Even though it may sound strange, dark chocolate can be a nutritious dessert option. Having been proved to have anti-cancer qualities, dark chocolate is abundant in antioxidants.

Sorbet made with fresh berries is a pleasant way to get your recommended daily intake of nutrients that fight cancer. Berries are another excellent source of antioxidants.

Parfait of yogurt: Yogurt's probiotic content can strengthen your immune system and lessen inflammation. A tasty and nutritious dessert can be created by layering yogurt with fruit and granola. Apples baked: Apples are rich in fiber and flavonoids, which are substances that fight cancer. A healthy and scrumptious dessert option can be made by baking apples with a dash of cinnamon.

Essentially, a healthy dessert should concentrate on whole, nutrient-dense foods that are low in sugar and bad fats. You can satisfy your sweet taste while simultaneously looking out for your health by selecting wise dessert choices.

There are other products and methods you can utilize to prepare sweets that are not only delectable but also cancer-fighting in addition to the healthy dessert options described above.
Here are some more suggestions for cooking nutritious sweets to avoid cancer.

Employ whole grains: For baking, use whole-grain flours as opposed to refined ones. Whole grains are rich in fiber and other nutrients that can lower the risk of cancer.

Including nuts and seeds: Nuts and seeds are a great source of fiber, healthy fats, and other nutrients that can help prevent cancer. Try using them as crusts, garnishes, or ingredients in your dessert dishes.

Choose low-sugar sweeteners because too much sugar can cause the body to become inflammatory, which has been linked to a higher risk of developing cancer. Use natural sweeteners like honey, maple syrup, or stevia as an alternative to conventional sugar.

Add spices: Several spices, including turmeric and ginger, have anti-inflammatory and cancer-preventing effects. If you want to add flavor and nutritional benefits to your desserts, try adding them.

Play around with plant-based ingredients: You can create decadent sweets that are both healthful and cancer-fighting by using foods like avocado, coconut milk, and tofu that are derived from plants.

You can enjoy sweets while promoting your health and lowering your risk of cancer by utilizing these suggestions and adding components that fight cancer to your desserts.

CHAPTER NINE

EXERCISE, STRESS MANAGEMENT, AND OTHER LIFESTYLE RECOMMENDATIONS FOR CANCER PREVENTION

The corpus of research on the influence of lifestyle variables on cancer prevention has been expanding in recent years. According to this research, altering one's lifestyle can significantly lower one's risk of developing cancer and can also be a main and secondary method of preventing the disease (preventing the recurrence of cancer in individuals who have already had the disease).

Millions of people worldwide are impacted by the deadly disease of cancer, and efforts to avoid it have been underway for decades. Changes in lifestyle have been demonstrated to lower the risk of acquiring cancer, while there is no surefire strategy to prevent the disease. "Lifestyle Recommendations for Cancer Prevention: Exercise, Stress Management, and More" covers some of the most important lifestyle modifications that can help prevent cancer.

One of the most crucial dietary modifications that can lower your risk of developing cancer is exercise. Many cancers, including breast, colon, and prostate cancer, have been proven to have a lower risk when regular exercise is undertaken. Inflammation can lead to the emergence of cancer and is reduced by exercise. The immune system may be strengthened as a result, aiding in the rejection of cancerous cells.

Stress reduction is a key lifestyle modification for cancer prevention together with exercise. Prolonged stress may increase the risk of cancer and impair the immune system, making it more challenging for the body to fight off cancer cells. Deep breathing, yoga, and other stress-reduction practices can help lower stress and enhance general health.

The prevention of cancer also depends on diet. Many types of cancer can be prevented by eating a balanced diet high in fruits, vegetables, whole grains, and lean protein. Nuts, berries, and leafy greens are examples of foods high in antioxidants that can help the body fight cancer-causing free radicals. Contrarily, a higher risk of cancer has been associated with the use of processed meals, red meat, and sugary beverages.
It is also essential for cancer prevention to avoid dangerous substances like smoke and excessive alcohol use. Smoking is connected to a number of cancers, including lung, bladder, and throat cancer, and is the main factor in deaths from cancer that could have been prevented. The chance of developing numerous cancers, including breast and liver cancer, has also been raised by excessive alcohol intake.

In order to prevent cancer, routine cancer screenings are crucial. At its earliest stages, when it is most treatable, cancer can be found via screening procedures including mammograms, colonoscopies, and Pap tests. The suggested screenings for a given age, family history, and other risk factors should be discussed with a healthcare professional.

Reducing chronic inflammation in the body is one of the main ways that changing one's lifestyle helps prevent cancer. A good diet and regular exercise have been found to lower the body's level of chronic inflammation, which is a known risk factor for a number of cancers. For instance, studies have indicated that exercise can lower blood levels of inflammatory indicators like C-reactive protein (CRP) and interleukin-6 (IL-6), while a diet rich in fruits and vegetables has been associated to lower levels of inflammatory markers like tumor necrosis factor-alpha (TNF-alpha).

Changes in lifestyle can lessen inflammation while also enhancing the immune system's performance, which is crucial for cancer prevention. While stress-reduction methods like yoga and meditation have been found to improve immune function by lowering stress levels in the body, regular exercise has been demonstrated to improve the immune system's capacity to detect and eliminate cancer cells.

Reducing exposure to environmental toxins and other carcinogens is another significant way that lifestyle changes can prevent cancer. Smoking is the main cause of lung cancer in the United States, and tobacco smoke, for instance, includes more than 70 recognized carcinogens. Those who stop smoking have a much lower risk of getting lung cancer as well as pancreatic, bladder, and cervical cancer.

Another lifestyle component, alcohol use, has been connected to a higher risk of numerous cancers, including esophageal, breast, and liver cancer. While severe drinking has been linked to an increased risk of cancer, moderate alcohol consumption—defined as up to one drink per day for women and up to two drinks per day for men—is usually seen to be safe.

Also important to the fight against cancer are dietary considerations. A diet high in red and processed meat, saturated fat, and added sugars has been linked to an increased risk of several types of cancer, including colon, pancreatic, and breast cancer, while a diet high in fruits, vegetables, whole grains, and lean protein has been linked to a lower risk of several types of cancer. Research has revealed that some foods and nutrients, like berries, leafy greens, and omega-3 fatty acids, may have particular cancer-preventive characteristics.

Cancer can be prevented in large part by modifying one's lifestyle, including regular exercise, stress reduction, a balanced diet, and abstaining from dangerous substances. Despite the fact that there is no surefire way to avoid cancer, including these lifestyle modifications into one's daily routine can help lower the risk of developing the disease while also enhancing general health and wellbeing. To create a personalized cancer prevention strategy based on each person's unique risk factors and health situation, people should collaborate with their healthcare professionals.

The maintenance of a healthy weight is also crucial for cancer prevention. Breast, colon, and prostate cancer have all been found to be more common in people who are obese. The risk of acquiring these cancers can be decreased by maintaining a healthy weight through a balanced diet and frequent exercise.

Lifestyle modifications like regular exercise, stress management, a balanced diet, avoiding dangerous substances, routine cancer screenings, and keeping a healthy weight can all help prevent cancer. The chance of acquiring cancer can be decreased and general health and wellbeing can be improved by following these actions, even though there is no 100% guarantee that cancer can be prevented.

CHAPTER TEN

DIETARY GUIDELINES TO PREVENT CANCER

A key component of cancer prevention is maintaining a balanced diet. Even though there is no way to completely eradicate the danger of cancer, adopting healthy eating habits can greatly lower the risk of getting cancer. To avoid cancer, follow these dietary recommendations:

Consume a variety of fruits and vegetables since they are high in vitamins, minerals, and antioxidants that help shield the body from cancer-causing agents. A variety of minerals and antioxidants that support a healthy immune system can be found in the colorful fruits and vegetables that you eat.

Steer clear of red and processed meats: These foods have been linked to an increased risk of colorectal and stomach cancer. Fish, chicken, beans, lentils, and tofu are all lean protein alternatives to these meats.

Reduce your alcohol intake because it has been linked to an increased risk of cancer, including breast, liver, and colorectal cancer. One drink for women per day and two for men per day should be the maximum alcohol intake to lower the risk of cancer.

Choose whole grains since they contain fiber, vitamins, and minerals that can lower the risk of cancer. Refined grains should not be substituted for whole-grain bread, pasta, or cereal.

Limit your sugar intake because it has been shown to increase inflammation, which has been related to a higher risk of cancer. Instead of drinking sugary beverages or eating sweet treats, choose entire fruits rather than fruit juice.

Consume healthy fats: Good fats, such those in nuts, seeds, avocados, and oily fish, can offer vital nutrients and guard against cancer. Limit saturated fats found in animal sources and steer clear of trans fats.

Be hydrated: Consuming plenty of water and other fluids can aid in the body's ability to rid itself of toxins, which lowers the risk of cancer. Make an effort to drink eight glasses of water each day.

To lower the risk of cancer, it's crucial to avoid smoking, maintain a healthy weight, and practice regular exercise in addition to the good dietary advice above. Your risk of getting cancer can be considerably decreased by adopting a healthy lifestyle, which can also enhance your general health and wellbeing.

Including cruciferous foods: Cruciferous vegetables, such as broccoli, cauliflower, cabbage, and kale, contain a substance called sulforaphane that has been demonstrated to have cancer-preventing qualities. These vegetables are also rich in fiber and other necessary elements.

Incorporate vitamin D sources: Vitamin D is a vital cancer preventative that many people do not receive enough of. Incorporate foods high in vitamin D in your diet, such as fatty fish, egg yolks, fortified milk, and orange juice. Sun exposure is another way to receive vitamin D, but be careful not to burn your skin.

Including herbs and spices: In addition to giving food taste, herbs and spices also offer anti-inflammatory and antioxidant characteristics that may help lower the risk of cancer. Spice up your meals using spices like cinnamon, ginger, and turmeric as well as herbs like basil, parsley, and thyme.

Choose foods with a low glycemic index to avoid blood sugar spikes, which can encourage inflammation and raise the risk of cancer. Foods with a high glycemic index, such as refined carbohydrates and sugar, can also induce these spikes. Go for foods with a low glycemic index, such as whole grains, legumes, and non-starchy vegetables.

Reduce your intake of processed and packaged foods because they frequently contain high levels of sugar, bad fats, and artificial additives that can raise your chance of developing cancer. As much as you can, choose whole, unprocessed foods; stay away from processed snacks and convenience foods.

You can lower your risk of cancer and enhance your general health and well-being by adopting a healthy diet and lifestyle. Also, keep in mind to get frequent cancer tests, maintain a healthy weight, and stay away from dangerous chemicals and substances.

CHAPTER ELEVEN

MEALS IDEAS THAT MAY HELP PREVENT CANCER

Quinoa And Roasted Veggies With Grilled Salmon

Ingredients:

1 salmon fillet
1 cup cooked quinoa
2 cups of mixed vegetables (broccoli, carrots, and bell peppers)
2 cloves garlic, minced
1 tablespoon olive oil
Salt and pepper to taste

Instructions:

200°C/400°F oven preheat.
Place the mixed vegetables in a single layer on a baking sheet, then sprinkle with olive oil. Add pepper and salt to taste.
The vegetables should be soft and slightly browned after roasting for 20 to 25 minutes.
A grill pan should be heated to medium-high heat while the vegetables are roasting. Add salt and pepper to the salmon fillet and grill for 3 to 4 minutes on each side, or until the salmon is well cooked. Olive oil and minced

garlic are heated over medium heat in a small saucepan until aromatic.

Together with quinoa and roasted veggies, serve the salmon over a grill. Garlic oil should be drizzled on top.

Chickpea And Spinach Curry

Ingredients:

1 can chickpeas, drained and rinsed
2 cups spinach leaves
1 onion, chopped
2 cloves garlic, minced
1 tablespoon grated ginger
1 tablespoon curry powder
1 can diced tomatoes
1 cup vegetable broth
Salt and pepper to taste

Instructions:

Heat some oil to a medium-high temperature in a big pot. When the onion is tender and transparent, add it and continue to cook.

When aromatic, add the curry powder, garlic, and ginger and simmer for an additional one to two minutes.

Bring to a simmer after adding the tomato-diced broth. The curry will thicken and the spinach will wilt after 10 to 15 minutes of simmering with the addition of the chickpeas and spinach.

According to taste, add salt and pepper.
Over quinoa or brown rice, plate the chickpea and
spinach curry.

Berry And Kale Smoothie

Ingredients:

1 cup frozen mixed berries
1 cup kale leaves
1 banana
1/2 cup plain Greek yogurt
1/2 cup almond milk
1 tablespoon honey (optional)

Instructions:

Blend all ingredients until they are smooth.
If desired, garnish the smoothie with extra berries or kale
leaves and serve right away.

Lentil And Vegetable Stir-fry

Ingredients:

1 cup brown lentils, cooked
2 cups mixed vegetables (broccoli, bell peppers, carrots,
onion)
2 cloves garlic, minced

1 tablespoon grated ginger
2 tablespoons soy sauce
1 tablespoon honey
1 tablespoon sesame oil
Salt and pepper to taste

Instructions:

A wok or big skillet over high heat should be used to warm the sesame oil.
For two to three minutes, stir-fry the mixed vegetables until they start to soften.
After one minute of stirring, add the ginger and garlic.
For a further two to three minutes, stir-fry the cooked lentils with the soy sauce and honey until well warm.
According to taste, add salt and pepper.
Over quinoa or brown rice, plate the lentil and vegetable stir-fry.

Grilled Chicken With Roasted Sweet Potatoes and brussels sprouts

Ingredients:

1 chicken breast
2 cups cubed sweet potatoes
2 cups halved Brussels sprouts
2 cloves garlic, minced
1 tablespoon olive oil

Salt and pepper to taste

Instructions:

Oven should be preheated to 400°F (200°C).
Place the Brussels sprouts and sweet potatoes on a
baking sheet, then sprinkle with olive oil. Use salt and
pepper to season.
Vegetables should be roasted for 20 to 25 minutes, or
until they are soft and just beginning to brown.
Heat a grill pan over medium-high heat while the
vegetables are roasting. Add salt and pepper to the
chicken breast and grill for 5 to 6 minutes on each side,
or until the chicken is thoroughly cooked.
Serve roasted Brussels sprouts and sweet potatoes
alongside the grilled chicken.

Spinach And Mushroom Omelette

Ingredients:

2 eggs
1 cup spinach leaves
1/2 cup sliced mushrooms
1/4 cup shredded cheddar cheese
Salt and pepper to taste

Instructions:

Mix the eggs with a fork in a small bowl. Put some pepper and salt for taste

A non-stick skillet is warmed up on medium. After adding, add the thinly sliced mushrooms and cook for two to three minutes, or until softened.

Sauté the spinach leaves for one more minute, or until they are wilted.

The bottom should be set after cooking the beaten eggs in the skillet for two to three minutes.

On one half of the omelette, scatter the cheddar cheese slices.

The other omelette half should be folded over the cheese using a spatula.

The eggs should be fully cooked and the cheese should be melted, which takes another minute.

the heated omelette with spinach and mushrooms.

Roasted Vegetable And Quinoa Salad

Ingredients:

1 cup cooked quinoa
2 cups mixed vegetables (zucchini, eggplant, red onion, bell peppers)
1 can chickpeas, drained and rinsed
2 tablespoons balsamic vinegar
2 tablespoons olive oil
Salt and pepper to taste

Instructions:

Oven should be heated to 400°F (200°C).
On a baking sheet, arrange the mixed veggies and
sprinkle with olive oil. Add salt and pepper to taste.
Vegetables should be roasted for 20 to 25 minutes or
until they are soft and slightly browned.
To make a dressing, combine the olive oil and balsamic
vinegar in a small bowl.
The cooked quinoa, roasted veggies, and chickpeas
should all be combined in a big bowl.
Toss salad with dressing after drizzling it over it.
add salt and pepper to the food for taste
The quinoa and roasted veggie salad should be served
at room temperature.

Grilled Tofu And Vegetable Skewers

Ingredients:

1 block firm tofu, cut into cubes
2 cups mixed vegetables (cherry tomatoes, zucchini, bell
peppers, mushrooms)
2 cloves garlic, minced
2 tablespoons olive oil
Salt and pepper to taste

Instructions:

Set the heat on the grill or grill pan to medium-high.

Vegetables in various combinations are skewered with tofu.

Garlic, olive oil, salt, and pepper should all be incorporated into a small bowl to form a marinate.

The skewers should be covered in the marinade.

The vegetables should be soft and slightly browned after grilling the skewers for 8 to 10 minutes, flipping them once.

Hot, with fresh herbs on top if preferred, serve the grilled tofu and veggie skewers

CHAPTER TWELVE

SMOOTHIES TO PREVENT CANCER

Here are some smoothie recipes with cancer-preventive ingredients that can be a part of a diet.

Blueberry And Almond Butter Smoothie

Ingredients:

1 cup frozen blueberries
1 banana
2 tablespoons almond butter
1 cup almond milk
1 teaspoon honey (optional)

Instructions:

Put all the ingredients in a blender, and blend until they are completely smooth.
With fresh blueberries or, if preferred, a drizzle of almond butter on top, serve the smoothie right away.

Green Tea and Berry Smoothie

Ingredients

1 cup brewed green tea, cooled
1 cup mixed berries (strawberries, blueberries, raspberries)
1/2 cup plain Greek yogurt
1 tbsp honey
1 cup ice
Blend all ingredients until smooth.

Turmeric And Ginger Smoothie

Ingredients

1 cup unsweetened almond milk
1/2 frozen banana
1/2 tsp turmeric
1/2 tsp grated ginger
1 tbsp chia seeds
1 cup spinach
Blend all ingredients until smooth.

Beet And Carrot Smoothie

Ingredients

1 cup beet juice
1/2 cup carrot juice
1/2 frozen banana
1/2 cup plain Greek yogurt
1/2 tsp cinnamon

1 cup ice
Blend all ingredients until smooth.

Kale And Mango Smoothie

Ingredients

1 cup unsweetened almond milk
1 cup kale leaves
1/2 cup frozen mango
1/2 frozen banana
1 tbsp honey
1 tbsp almond butter
Blend all ingredients until smooth.

Blueberry And Flaxseed Smoothie

Ingredients

1 cup unsweetened almond milk
1 cup frozen blueberries
1 tbsp ground flaxseed
1/2 cup plain Greek yogurt
1/2 tsp vanilla extract
1 cup ice
Blend all ingredients until smooth.

Pineapple And Turmeric Smoothie

Ingredients

1 cup unsweetened almond milk
1 cup frozen pineapple
1/2 tsp turmeric
1/2 tsp grated ginger
1/2 cup plain Greek yogurt
1 tbsp honey
Blend all ingredients until smooth.

Berry And Avocado Smoothie

Ingredients

1 cup unsweetened almond milk
1 cup mixed berries (strawberries, blueberries, raspberries)
1/2 avocado
1/2 cup plain Greek yogurt
1 tbsp honey
1 cup ice
Blend all ingredients until smooth.

Chocolate And Peanut Butter Smoothie

Ingredients

1 cup unsweetened almond milk
1/2 frozen banana
1 tbsp cocoa powder
1 tbsp natural peanut butter

1/2 tsp vanilla extract
1 cup ice
Blend all ingredients until smooth.

Carrot And Orange Smoothie

Ingredients

1 cup carrot juice
1/2 cup freshly squeezed orange juice
1/2 frozen banana
1/2 cup plain Greek yogurt
1 tbsp honey
1 cup ice
Blend all ingredients until smooth.

Spinach And Mango Smoothie

Ingredients

1 cup unsweetened almond milk
1 cup spinach
1/2 cup frozen mango
1/2 frozen banana
1 tbsp honey
1 tbsp chia seeds
Blend all ingredients until smooth.

These smoothies aren't meant to take the place of
medical care or guidance. Before changing your diet,
please speak with your doctor or a trained nutritionist.